An Introduction to the Study of the Mind

By Walter Scott Athearn
Director School of Religious Education and
Social Service, Boston University

Being Section Three of
"Teaching the Teacher"

Copyright © 2017 Read Books Ltd.
This book is copyright and may not be
reproduced or copied in any way without
the express permission of the publisher in writing

British Library Cataloguing-in-Publication Data
A catalogue record for this book is available from the
British Library

Contents

I. What Is the Mind?..	147
II. The Machine and the Machinist	150
III. The Triune Man..	154
IV. The Intellect..	157
V. The Emotions...	160
VI. The Will...	163
VII. Habit Formation.......................................	166
VIII. How to Study..	170
IX. The Growing Mind.....................................	173
X. Workers with Immortal Souls	176

LESSON I
What Is the Mind?

The Question Answered. "What is mind?" inquired a student of a great teacher. "No matter," came the answer promptly. "But," continued the student, "what is matter?" Whereupon the famous teacher answered simply, "Never mind." An inspired writer recorded the dual nature of man in these words: "And Jehovah God formed man of the dust of the ground, and breathed into his nostrils the breath of life; and man became a living soul." What is this "living soul" which is not "dust of the ground"? It is that something which **thinks** and **feels** and **wills**. Mind, like electricity, is defined by describing its behavior. How does mind behave? It thinks and feels and wills.

All that we know about the mind is called psychology; all that we know about plants is called botany; all that we know about animal life is called zoölogy; all that we know about the starry heavens is called astronomy. Psychology is the science of mind and its behavior. Mind is that which thinks and feels and wills.

The Attributes of the Mind. Can we say anything about mind except that it thinks and feels and wills? It has already been pointed out that mind is **immaterial**; it is not matter. Matter obeys the law of gravitation; it has weight. Matter obeys the law of inertia; its direction is determined by objects or forces outside of itself; it cannot start until something starts it, and it cannot stop until something stops it. But mind does not obey the law of gravitation; it has no weight and it does not fall toward the center of the earth when a physical support is removed. Neither does mind obey the law of inertia; it is not stopped and started by physical forces or objects outside of itself. Mind does not obey the laws of matter; mind is immaterial. The mind has four other attributes which succeeding paragraphs will describe. Besides being **immaterial**, the mind is **unitary, self-active, self-conscious, and abiding.**

The Mind Is Unitary. The mind that thinks is the mind that feels; the mind that thinks and feels is the mind that wills. These three activities are kinds of behavior of one mind. We do not have three minds; we have but one mind which does three different things. The mind is **unitary**. When the mind is thinking, it cannot be devoting its entire energy to feeling or willing. We have only one hundred per cent of mental energy. If eighty per cent is engaged in thinking, there will be only twenty per cent which can be used for feeling and willing. If ninety per cent is engaged in feeling only ten per cent will remain for thinking and willing. Students cannot study well when they are in a state of emotional tension. There is little use to reason with a stubborn child while the will is dominating the mental life. Parents and teachers should remember that every mental state has a direct bearing on other mental states. There is but one mind—it can think and feel and will, but it has but one hundred per cent of mental energy to distribute among these activities at any one time.

The Mind Is Self-Active. A stone thrown into the air will continue to move until it is drawn back to earth by the force of gravitation. It has no power to start or stop itself or to change its own direction. But the mind is **self-active**. It can change its own behavior; it can initiate or discontinue various directions of activity.

The Mind Is Self-Conscious. An old German philosopher gave a great dinner to celebrate the first occasion on which his baby boy said "I." "That act," said the philosopher, "proves that my boy is a human being." The human mind says "I." It is conscious of its own behavior. It not only thinks and feels and wills, but it says, "I think," "I feel," "I will." The steam engine moves, but it does not know that it moves. The mind is conscious of its own behavior.

The Mind Is Abiding. When a lighted match touches a piece of paper, the paper burns. Its chemical structure is changed. The paper ceases to exist as paper. It has been changed into smoke and ashes. There is as much matter in the world as there was before the paper was burned, but there is less paper. **Matter** is indestructible, but **paper** is not. Matter, modified, loses its identity. But the mind passes through all the myriad changes of human experience from the cradle to the grave without losing its identity. Matter, modified, **loses** its identity; mind, modified, **retains** its identity. Mind is **immortal**.

I Am Always I, and You Are Always You. One summer day, more than forty years ago, when the writer was a very small boy, he wandered out into the spacious yard which surrounded his boyhood home. He soon discovered a rain barrel beneath the eaves of the house. Childish curiosity prompted him to push a broken chair beside the barrel and then to climb upon the chair so that he could look into the barrel. The barrel was nearly full of water. The sun was shining in such manner as to produce a perfect image of the boy in the water.

I put my hand down to the image, and the image put its hand up to me. Soon I was completely absorbed in delightful play with the image in the barrel. While I was thus engaged, my big brother slipped up behind me, lifted my feet from the chair, and pushed me head-first into the barrel of water. I gave one loud, terrified scream before my head went under the water and then down, down, down I went. It seemed to me that I should never touch the bottom. I can remember, vividly, what I thought as I descended into that rain barrel. My first thought was, "I wonder if I can swallow it all?" My next thought was, "Shall I never reach the bottom?" Just then my mother, who had heard my scream, caught me by the heels and pulled me, dripping, from the barrel. How well I remember the feeling of anger which filled my mind as I discovered my brother hiding behind the rain barrel and realized that it was he who had caused my unexpected descent into the barrel! And I remember also the thrill of joy that filled my soul when my mother spanked my brother for "ducking" me.

Over forty years have passed since my rain-barrel experience, yet the same "I" who was "ducked" in that rain barrel is penning these lines in which all the feelings and volitions and thoughts of the event are vividly recalled. I have passed through joys and sorrows, I have traveled many, many miles, my mind has had the discipline of years in schools and colleges, and yet I am the same "I" of my childhood days. I have been modified by the experience of a busy life, but I have retained my identity.

But while the same "I" that was "ducked" in the rain barrel so long ago is here to-day, not an atom of the body of the boy who was "ducked" in the rain barrel is here now. I have lived in several different bodies since that childhood experience. The shifting chemical atoms of my body have come and gone, but I have remained "I" through all the years. I am a modified "I," but still the same "I." I was "I" in a body of fifty pounds; I was "I" in a body of one hundred pounds; now as a grown man I am still "I" in a body of one hundred and sixty pounds. Cut off my arms, and I am "I"; cut off my legs, and I am still "I." Mutilate my body as you may and I shall still be "I." And when my body shall crumble into dust I shall still be the abiding, "immortal I" which even death cannot destroy. What a sublime thought it is that **I am always I, and you are always you!** Matter modified loses its identity, but mind modified retains its identity.

Summary

Mind is that which thinks and feels and wills. Mind has five attributes. It is immaterial. It is unitary. It is self-active. It is self-conscious. It is abiding or immortal. The science which deals with the mind and its behavior is called psychology.

Questions for Review

1. Define mind.
2. Define psychology.
3. Name five attributes of mind and describe each.
4. Give an example from your own experience which illustrates the unity of mind.
5. If mind is self-active, can the teacher determine just how the pupil will interpret the facts presented in the curriculum? Is the child's mind simply a vessel to be filled?
6. Discuss the influence of early impressions on the abiding mind.

LESSON II
The Machine and the Machinist

The Dust of the Earth. If a chemist should analyze the human body he would find in it sixteen chemical elements. His analysis would reveal carbon, oxygen, hydrogen, sulphur, and a dozen other chemicals. In the body of the average-sized man the chemist would find enough iron to make a spike big enough to hang a man upon; he would find enough lead to make seven hundred and eighty dozen lead pencils; enough phosphorus to make the heads for twenty-two hundred dozen matches, enough illuminating gas to inflate a balloon which would carry a man into the air. He would find two pounds of lime, twenty spoonfuls of salt, and sixty lumps of sugar, besides hydrochloric acid and other chemicals in smaller quantities.

If the same chemist should analyze a quantity of the "dust of the ground" he would find about seventy different chemical elements. If he should write in two parallel columns the seventy chemical elements found in the "dust of the ground" and the sixteen chemical elements found in man he would find that all of the chemical elements in man's body are found among the seventy elements in the "dust of the ground." The simple facts compel us to say that some great chemist took from the seventy elements in the "dust of the ground" sixteen elements and fashioned them into man's body.

If the same chemist should analyze one thousand hen's eggs he would find almost exactly the same distribution of chemical elements as in man's body. Is a man nothing but one thousand hen's eggs? Is he nothing but nails and lead and salt and sugar and illuminating gas?

A Living Soul. But there is something about a man which eludes the chemist. The delicately attuned apparatus which detects and photographs chemical substances in planets millions of miles away, or which penetrates flesh and bone and reveals the structure of hidden tissue, cannot record the growth of ideals in the mind of a child or the emotions and volitions which stir the hearts of men. No, the chemical laboratory cannot reveal the mind of man. Another kind of laboratory has been established for this purpose. It is the **psychological** laboratory. The presence of the psychological laboratory is conclusive evidence that man is more than "dust of the ground." By some wonderful process man became "a living soul." I **am** "a living soul," but I **have** a body which is "dust of the ground."

The Human Machine. Considered as a machine, man's body is a marvelous combination of chemical, physical, and biological properties. It is, indeed, a wonderful "temple of clay" for the soul of man. To understand his body, man must study deeply into the science of chemistry, into physiology and anatomy; he must know the laws of growth and the facts of heredity. This knowledge is necessary if man is to keep his body a fit dwelling place for his spirit.

The Nervous System. The nervous system is the seat of the mental life. The human soul may be said to dwell in the midst of the nervous system, not as a captive awaiting a day of liberation, but as a master using the wonderful apparatus for his own ends. The brain and spinal cord with a multitude of sensory and motor nerves constitute what is known as the **central nervous system.** The brain is the central office from which all mental life emanates. This central office is connected with the outside world by thousands of nerves, telegraphic wires, which carry into the central office messages of every kind. Besides these sensory nerves which keep the mind informed regarding the outside world, the mind has the service of another group of nerves, called the motor nerves, which carry messages from the brain to all parts of the body.

In the midst of the nervous system sits the mind, the immortal "I," like a telegraph operator interpreting the dots and dashes that constantly pour in over many wires from the ends of the earth, and, with fingers on the key, sending answering messages which change the course of human history. As I write these words I am on an island in the midst of the sea. Save for my wife there is not another human being for miles in any direction. My auditory nerves carry to my mind the surge of the waves against the rock-bound coast; my olfactory nerves bring the odor of the pines on the cliff above me; my optical nerves bring me the gorgeous hues of yellow, orange, and red of a beautiful August sunset. But suppose there should suddenly cross the horizon the outline of a dozen canoes rapidly propelled by painted savages. As they grow nearer weapons are revealed by their sides. They approach our island; they grasp their weapons and prepare to land. Suppose that this has been revealed to me by my sensory nerves. Must I sit here motionless and let these savages kill my wife and myself? No, the "immortal I" has the use of another set of nerves. A message goes out to my motor nerves. Arms and legs and tongue are in action. We seek safety.

The Machinist. Man does not need to be damned by his environment. He has the power to change his environment. He learns from his sensory nerves what his environment is; if this environment does not suit him, he has the power to move to another environment or to change his present environment. The mind of man, the self, the "immortal I," has power to have dominion over the earth.

Suppose, for example, that a young man finds himself a member of a group or "gang" of young men who swear, smoke, and chew tobacco, desecrate the Sabbath Day, idle away their time, and whose ideals are low and unworthy. Must the young man remain a member of this group and conform to its standards? No, this young man can say to his legs: "Legs, get me out of this gang. Take me over to the Christian Endeavor Society. Take me to the Bible class. Take me to the Y. M. C. A. Get me away from this environment." It is the mind of the young man, not his muscles or his nervous system, which issues the command to move into a new environment or to change the old associations. Man, the machinist, is the architect of his own fate, the determiner of his own destiny.

The Chart and Compass. How shall the mind of man, the "immortal I," know how to guide him amidst the conflicting interests and ideals of this life? Has he no chart or compass? In his inner soul, if man will but listen, he can hear the voice of conscience, the captain of his fate, guiding him into paths of safety. At his hand he finds a guidebook, the Holy Bible, telling him that he is made in the image of the Father and commissioning him to "subdue" the earth. In this Book he learns the story of his Elder Brother, who is his perfect Pattern, his infallible Guide, and Saviour. In a world of sin and suffering he hears the command to go forth and make all things new. "Go ye into all the world!" What a divine calling for the "immortal I"!

Summary

Man is a living soul; he has a body which is dust of the earth. The body is man's servant. Through it he learns the facts about the physical universe, and with it he adjusts himself to the world in which he lives or makes the world over to conform to his ideals. Man is not the slave of his environment. He may conquer environment. He will study chemistry, physiology, anatomy, and biology that he may know the laws which govern his body, but he will study the Bible, and especially the life of Christ, that he may know the laws which govern the life of his immortal spirit.

Questions for Review and Discussion

1. What evidence is there that man is dust of the earth?
2. What fact does the erection of psychological laboratories establish?
3. Give a brief discussion of the function of the central nervous system.
4. Give illustrations from your own experience of how men and women have overcome unfortunate environment.
5. What function has the Church in determining the environment of people?
6. What is the standard for human conduct?
7. Who is responsible for teaching this standard to the "immortal I's" who are to have dominion over the earth?

LESSON III
The Triune Man

Man, a Triune Being. Man thinks and feels and wills. In his mental life the "immortal I," of which we have been thinking, is a triune being. The following diagram will show man's threefold mental life:

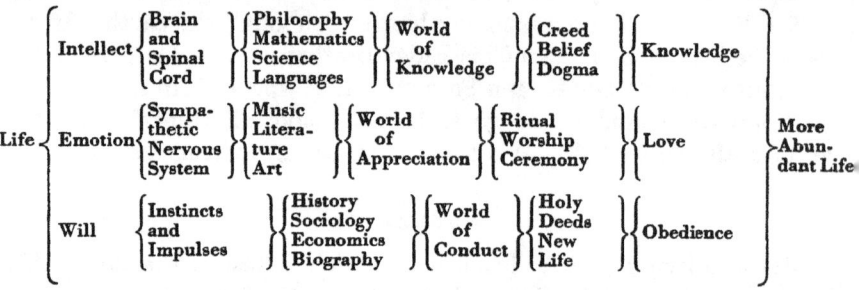

Control Through Intellect. One of man's chief sources of controlling, modifying, and regulating his conduct is his **intellect**. Intellect operates through the brain and spinal cord. Through this physical means of approach man develops his intellect by the study of such disciplines as philosophy, mathematics, sciences, and foreign languages. Through the intellect man comes to live in **a world of knowledge.** His mind is stored with facts and ideas. When man takes his intellect into the field of religion it gives him knowledge about God. This is the source of religious creeds, beliefs, dogma.

Control Through Emotions. A second method of control is through the emotions. The emotions, besides calling upon the brain and spinal cord, depend upon the sympathetic nervous system. The emotions are developed by such studies as music, art, and literature. This gives one **a world of appreciation.** Besides knowing things with the intellect, man attaches to the things he knows certain values which his intellect cannot know. When one takes his emotions into religion it gives rise to worship, to ritual, and to ceremonies. The emotions provide affection and love in religion.

Control Through Will. A third method of control is through the will. The will calls into play the deep-seated instincts and impulses in one's biological nature. We discipline the will in the schools through the study of history, sociology, economics, and biography.

This gives us a world of conduct. In the realm of religion the will gives us the religious deed, visiting the sick, giving a cup of water "in his name."

"Lopsided" People. When one uses but one of his three faculties for control it leaves him "lopsided." The absent-minded mathematician may lose all interest in the harmony of sound or the balance in color combination just because he has failed to develop his world of appreciation. He becomes an intellectual "freak." In religion a man may develop great skill in dogmatic disputes, and fail to appreciate the emotional values in the great concepts which he defends with such rigid logic. Such a man is a religious "freak."

The musician or painter may cultivate his emotional nature at the expense of his world of knowledge and his world of conduct. We excuse him by saying that it is "artistic temperament," but we know that he is "lopsided." The emotionally lopsided man in the realm of religion is the "Holy Roller," the dancing dervish, the emotional religious freak.

One may also be lopsided in the direction of his will. He may be always acting before he thinks or without appreciating the emotional values involved in his deeds. In the realm of religion this gives us the man who tries to save himself by his good deeds. Such a man often says, "I care not what a man believes. I am only interested in what he does." All such are "lopsided."

Living in Three Worlds. The "balanced" man lives in three worlds—the world of knowledge, the world of appreciation, and the world of conduct. In our schools and colleges there arose a system of "majors" and "minors" to protect students from a one-sided development. If students selected their "majors" in the field of the intellect they were required to select a minor in the field of the emotions, and a second minor in the field of the will. If the major was selected in music, art, and literature, a minor must be selected in mathematics, science, language, or philosophy and a second minor in such subjects as history, biography, sociology, and economics.

The world has lopsided religions. Some say that religion is dogma and they try to save the world by knowledge only. Others say that religion is ritual and they prescribe ceremony and form as a means of salvation. Still others say that religion is good works and they neglect religious knowledge and ceremony. The "balanced" mind needs a religion which is **knowledge** and **ritual** and **deed.**

The Religion of Whole-Mindedness. Christianity is the religion of whole-mindedness. It has knowledge about God for one's intellect; love and worship of God for one's emotions; obedience to God for one's will. If the mind of man is to be fully satisfied with its religion, there must be regular study of God's truth for the intellect; systematic worship of God for the emotions; and constant service of God for the will. Failing in any one of these activities man's spiritual nature tends to starve, or to become partial and incomplete.

A Triune Man Needs a Triune God. We have seen that man is by nature a triune being. He is one; yet he is three. He is a thinker, a feeler, and a doer. He comes into being with this threefold nature hungering for development. The schools develop the mental capacity through science, art, and the humanities. But the complete fulfillment of man's being can come only through a religion which provides a triune God whom one may know, whom one may love, whom one may obey. The triune man is completed, through faith and love and obedience, by a triune God. A child begins life with a triune capacity for growth; through the Christian religion he may come to have life more abundantly.

Summary

Man has a threefold mental capacity. His mental balance requires the harmonious development of all his powers. Man may become mentally one-sided if any one of his mental powers is developed at the expense of other powers. There are mental "freaks" in all walks of life—religion is no exception to the rule. A "balanced" religious life requires discipline of the whole mind. Some of the world's religions feed the intellect only; some minister only to the emotions; and some provide only a program of good deeds. Christianity provides for the entire mental life and may truly be called "the religion of whole-mindedness."

Questions for Review and Discussion

1. Reproduce the diagram given in the first paragraph of this chapter.
2. Name and discuss briefly the three worlds in which all people should live.
3. State some ways in which people may become mentally "lopsided."
4. Recall some lopsided people and try to explain the cause of their lack of balance.

5. Enumerate your own religious practices and try to predict the effect of your present religious life on your own religious balance in years to come.
6. Explain why Christianity can claim to be the religion of whole-mindedness.

LESSON IV
The Intellect

The Faculties of the Intellect. The intellect is a name for the mind's capacity to think. For purposes of analysis the process of thinking is broken up into six faculties, as follows: Perception, Memory, Imagination, Conception, Judgment, and Reason. This chapter will attempt only a brief definition of these six faculties.

Perception. The telegraph operator sits at his desk and translates into messages the dots and dashes that flash from his instrument. The dots and dashes are raw material out of which messages are made. Just so the mind sits in the citadel of man's brain and translates into knowledge the raw material which comes pouring in from a thousand nerves. Sensations of sound, color, taste, smell, and touch are recorded in a multitude of combinations and with varying degrees of intensity. The mind's capacity to interpret these combinations into knowledge is called perception. Perception may be defined as the mind's capacity to **translate sensations into knowledge.** A simple message, the mind's impression of a single object, is called a **percept.**

It is the function of perception to store the mind with knowledge in the form of percepts. The richer the experience of the child— the wider the travel, the more varied the contact with nature, people, music, art, and literature—the greater will be the number and variety of percepts which can later be woven into the thought life of the adult.

Memory. Memory is the mind's power **to record, to retain, to recall,** and **to recognize** previous mental experiences. These four powers are sometimes referred to as the four R's of memory. There are laws governing each of these powers which the successful teacher should know. Laws of **attention** and **emotional preference** will determine how vividly the record is impressed; laws of **association** and **repetition** will determine how easily it will be recalled.

The primary law of memory may be stated in these words: **Things** held before the mind at the same time will tend to suggest each other. In other words, things that are experienced together will tend to be recalled together. This is the law of **association.** There are secondary laws of memory which every teacher and student should know. If things are frequently held in the mind together they will be more apt to suggest each other. This is the law of **repetition.** If the association of objects or ideas is attended by pleasurable emotion they will be more apt to be recalled together. This is the law of **emotional preference.** If some logical relationship can be discovered between two or more facts or ideas they will be more apt to be recalled together.

Imagination. Some one has aptly said that "Imagination is the mind's power of painting pictures without the present help of the senses." Perception stores the mind with raw material in the form of percepts. Memory recalls the past impressions to consciousness. Imagination picks up these recalled images and weaves them into new combinations the like of which no one has ever seen or heard before. When imagination works without a plan and images flit before the mind promiscuously it is **dreaming,** but when imagination works with a plan it builds its castles in the air with a purpose. It gives the architect his plan, the author his plot, the scientist his hypothesis. To man's religious life imagination gives the power to see reality in the realms of faith rather than in the material world.

Conception. The mind has the power to **digest** its experiences. Sensations coming in through eyes, ears, nose, and the other senses were first interpreted by perception into ideas of individual things, called percepts. But the mind has the power of refining percepts. The sensations of color, size, form, odor, which entered into the idea of the first apple, for example, are subjected to critical analysis. The mind discovers that an apple does not need to be red, or sour, or soft. After analyzing many apples the mind gets an idea of a **class of objects** which it will call apples. This idea is not a mental picture of any one apple; it is a definition of a term which will fit all apples. This definition is a concept. It is the mind's idea of a class of objects. The concept "apple" will hold many particular apples; the concept "horse" is a definition which will include all horses; the concept "boy" will include Tom, Dick, Harry, and all other individuals belonging to the boy class.

When the mind can think in terms of concepts it is able to think in mental shorthand—one word has become the symbol of many experiences. A concept, therefore, is the mind's idea of a class of objects, and conception is the mind's capacity to think in terms of concepts.

Judgment. Thinking is comparing. Comparing percepts produces concepts. **Comparing concepts produces judgments.** Iron and metal are both concepts. When I compare these two concepts and announce my conclusion, I say, "**Iron is a metal.**" This simple declarative sentence is a judgment.

Reason. Reasoning is **a comparison of judgments.**
First judgment: All men are mortal.
Second judgment: This person is a man.
Third judgment, resulting from comparing the first and second judgments: This person is mortal.

This process is called reasoning. The first judgment is usually called the **major premise**; the second judgment is called the **minor premise**; and the third or resulting judgment is called the **conclusion.** **Logic** is the name of the science which treats of the laws governing the process of reasoning.

Summary

There are six faculties of the intellect. The first translates sensations into ideas; the second recalls to the mind both the sensation and the idea; the third enlarges, modifies, and reconstructs images and ideas previously formed; the fourth refines images into definitions; the fifth enables the mind to think in terms of definitions; and the sixth enables the mind to think in terms of judgments.

Questions for Review and Discussion

1. Name the six faculties of the intellect.
2. Define the terms perception and percept.
3. Name the four R's of memory.
4. Repeat the primary law of memory.
5. Name two secondary laws of memory.
6. Define imagination.
7. Tell the difference between a percept and a concept.
8. Define judgment.
9. Define reason.

LESSON V
The Emotions

Emotions Defined. Emotion is a name for the mind's capacity to feel. We often use the term **feeling** when the experience is simple and less intense and apply the term **emotion** when the experience is more complex and more intense. The difference between feeling and emotion is in intensity, not in quality. Emotion is **personal** and **particular**. It is **my** pleasure and **my** pain, **my** happiness and **my** sorrow. Emotion is accompanied by physical or bodily behavior, but it is something more than physical; it is essentially a mental experience.

Kinds of Emotion. There are two kinds of emotion: the **egoistic** and the **altruistic**. The egoistic emotion flows in toward the self and makes the self the center of the experience. Like, dislike, reverence, love, friendship, tenderness, terror, hate, scorn, pride, vanity, and shame are among the **egoistic** emotions.

The **altruistic** emotions flow out from oneself toward others. Sharing happiness with others is altruistic. Pity is unhappiness through shared unhappiness. Malice is happiness through another's unhappiness. Envy is unhappiness through another's happiness.

Both kinds of emotions may be social or nonsocial, depending on whether or not the objects of the emotions are personal or nonpersonal. Among the nonsocial emotions are like and dislike applied to impersonal objects, æsthetic pleasure, logical pleasure, sense of humor, and the like.

The World of Appreciation. Emotion adds personal values to objects. The cottage on the hillside may have little intrinsic, commercial value, but if it is my boyhood home, around which memories of childhood cling, it will have an added meaning and value for me which is not fictitious, but very real. **Emotion** is more than an appraiser of values; it **creates values**. These values, created by emotion, give us our **world of appreciation**.

The Uses of Emotion. Emotion is a potent factor in the control of conduct. In the first place, it aids the individual to self-realization, fosters personal relationships, and gives a sense of the reality of other persons. In the second place, it tends to make one responsive to his environment and enables him to get higher personal values out of his surroundings. In the third place, it tends to break up habitual mental and bodily habits by its discovery of new values and its insistent demand that conduct shall be changed in recognition of these new values. In the fourth place, emotion, by breaking up old associations and by discovering new compelling interests, enables the mind to reorganize itself around the larger personality which religion furnishes and unites the smaller with the larger self. Thus emotion helps to unite the life of man with the life of God.

Expression and Growth. The emotions grow through expression. In harmony with the nature of all conscious states emotion tends to find expression in conduct. If normal expression in some form does not follow an emotional state one of two results is sure to appear sooner or later in the life of the individual: either serious nervous and mental disease involving "suppressed emotions" which derange the whole mental life, or the loss of the desire or ability to act on future emotional suggestions.

Excessive theater-going or novel-reading may prove very injurious to the mental life. Even the constant appeal of great religious interests, such as missionary, philanthropic, and social-service challenges, with no active response to the emotional demands, may cause one to lose the capacity to be aroused by future appeals. The heart is hardened by the denial of response, and the mental life has lost a capacity for response—an "unpardonable sin" has been committed. "The remedy would be," said Professor James, "never to suffer oneself to have an emotion without expressing it afterwards in some active way."

Rules for Control. The quotation from Professor James in the preceding paragraph advised that all emotional states should find expression **"in some active way."** This must not be interpreted to mean that all emotional desires should be gratified. There are emotional desires which should not be gratified, but something positive should be done with them. One of the pressing tasks before religious educators to-day is to organize a body of wholesome activities through which the emotional responses of youth may find safe and satisfying expression.

Five rules may aid in avoiding the dangers of undirected emotional response: 1. **The emotional response should be positive.** A conscious attempt to do a positive thing is much more effective than an effort to inhibit or suppress some undesirable tendency by sheer force of will power. The theory of casting out evil by doing good is still valid. 2. **Pleasurable responses should be encouraged.** There are pleasurable responses which are not desirable, but they are unde-

sirable for other reasons than their pleasurable qualities. Find substitutes which are equally desirable and which do not have the unwholesome attachments. Happy, hopeful, pleasing, courageous responses which challenge the mind's capacity to appreciate the good, the true, and the beautiful, are the types of emotional response most worth while.
3. **The altruistic responses should be encouraged.** The egoistic responses can usually be depended upon to take care of themselves. The altruistic responses enable us to share the experiences of others, thus enlarging our sympathies and expanding our personalities and increasing our powers both to give and to get pleasure and service. 4. **The emotional life should have a balanced development.** Music, art, literature, social response, æsthetic contemplation, logical pleasure, good humor—all these should have their place in the development of an emotional nature which is to serve the highest interests of the religious soul. 5. **A serious desire to be socially and remedially helpful should attend all reference to unwholesome emotional situations.** Sensational novels and problem plays are often filled with the most revolting scenes. They are defended on the ground that they express life as it is and that such literature adds to the completeness of experience. Miss Calkins, in "A First Book in Psychology," aptly quotes the following editorial from the Nation in condemnation of current tendencies to revive unpleasant emotions to no good purpose: "Their revelations of the hideous conditions of life are not calculated to make any person of good will seek out that suffering and relieve it. . . . In a time when sensationalism and overemphasis of all kinds bid fair to be regarded as the chief literary virtues, these sordid infernos go a step farther and deal consciously in the revolting. . . . To view a brutal action may be salutary if it prompts one to knock the brute down; to penetrate the lowest human depths, bearing aid, is well; to classify a new gangrene is well if it evokes a remedy: but to pray about a pathological laboratory that one may experience the last qualm of disgust and then to exploit such disgust for literary purposes, is to create a public nuisance."

Summary

Emotion is the mind's capacity to feel. It is personal and particular. There are two major groups of emotions, egoistic and altruistic. Emotions create new values and build our world of appreciation. Emotions serve (1) to foster self-realization; (2) to draw personal values out of the surroundings; (3) to break up the habitual mental life, and (4) to enlarge the personal life and unite it with the life of God. Emotions grow by expression and sicken and die when unexpressed. Wholesome development should be guided by rules which recognize the laws of the mental life. Five such rules are discussed in this chapter.

Questions for Review and Discussion

1. Define emotion.
2. Name the two major groups of emotions and give examples of each.
3. In what way does emotion add to the facts of experience?
4. Name and discuss four uses of emotion.
5. Discuss the paragraph on "Expression and Growth."
6. Give the five rules for the control of emotions.

LESSON VI

The Will

The Will Defined. Will is a name for **the mind's power to act**. Like emotion, will is personal. It ties persons and things to itself. In an act of will the mind conceives itself as having dominion over other selves or other objects. The will is the personal self conscious of its power over its environment. It moves everything else to suit its own purposes. It transforms people and things to its own ends. A dominant will gives a city a new charter; pushes a railroad across the plains; spans the surging stream with a suspension bridge; overcomes a malignant pestilence; develops a new cosmic theory; proposes a league of nations; expounds and champions a new religion. In every case the mind of man has acted on other minds and has led them to conform to a single will.

Forms of Will. Acts of the will may be **involuntary** or spontaneous; or they may be the result of deliberation and choice. In this latter case they are said to be **voluntary**. In the involuntary acts the will does not seem to refer its acts to any time or place. It seems to rest content in the exercise of its power over its objects without thought as to purpose or results. These acts are basic and more fundamental than the more deliberative acts of will. The second form of will, the voluntary act, is directed toward some future object or event.

If it hesitates in making its choices it is because two or more future ends present themselves for consideration, and time is consumed in weighing the pros and cons presented by each claimant before the final choice is made.

The Choice of Ends. Voluntary acts are choices of ends. The more vivid and definite the end, the more unhesitatingly will the choice be made. Three qualities characterize the ends for which will strives. 1. The end is **real**. There is no incentive to the will in a fictitious object. 2. It is always in the **future**. 3. It is always thought of as **dependent on the act of will**. A real, future event or person or object which the will can affect or influence is necessary to induce the will to act.

The disciplined will fixes its attention on the end to be attained, and lets the minor details adjust themselves automatically. The untrained will must give its attention to the details of adjustment until they have become involuntary. Smaller adjustments which are essential to a larger end tend to become automatic as soon as they are willed.

A young man wills to become a lawyer. He sees before him the clear-cut image of himself in future days as a trained attorney-at-law. If his will is disciplined, the adjustments necessary to realize the goal will be made without conscious effort. If he is not trained he will have consciously to will to attend college, to study Latin, to work during vacations for the necessary fees, or anything else which may be a prerequisite to the practice of law. After once willing to do any or all of these things necessary to become a lawyer, they will **tend** to become automatic and finally they will be performed without conscious effort.

Great men live simple lives. They make their life choices in terms of great fundamental purposes. Abraham Lincoln in the White House at Washington made his decisions in terms of the simple but fundamental rules that governed his life as a country lawyer in Illinois. Great and basic principles as ends in life tend to simplify all of life's decisions. Two simple rules should guide in the training of the will: **1. Select great, fundamental, worth-while ends for your life. 2. Will to do all the smaller things that are worthy means to the larger ends**

Faith and Belief. Will is **egoistic**. Faith is **altruistic**. When will turns from itself as the center, and sees some other person or object as the dominating, controlling force, then will has become lost in faith. The dominating will, master of all it surveys, suddenly sees in some other person qualities which command respect and obedience. From the "captain" of his own soul, a man quickly becomes the loyal subject of a loved and trusted leader. One has faith in a person: in his father, his teacher, his general, his God.

Or, the assertive will may see a worthy object in an impersonal truth or principle. This attitude of the will toward an impersonal object is belief. One believes in tariff legislation, in a league of nations, in a theory of the inspiration of the Bible.

Dominating Altruism. When the dominating, aggressive will finds a person or an object to whom it surrenders its power and to whom it renders loyal allegiance, it does not lose its forceful, aggressive attributes and become a passive, nonresisting state of mind. On the contrary, it retains all its militant aggressiveness. But its powers are no longer devoted to impressing its own will upon others; it now bends all its energies to the promotion of the will of the one to whom it has surrendered its own leadership. It now loyally loses itself in the life of another, and has a sense of finding a larger life in the act of losing a smaller life.

The Surrendered Life. "I surrender all," sings the Christian. But this surrender is but a transfer of **myself and my plans** as an end in life to **Christ and his plans for my life.** My own aggressive personality goes with me to the new life. In conquest I carry the will of Christ to the unconquered savage in the heart of Africa; with heroic courage I face the corruption in civic life and fasten Christ's will on a great city; with militant faith I enter the marts of trade and bid Capital and Labor follow the Man of Galilee; with high courage I give up my own plans for a selfish life and teach little children to "will to do the Father's will." The "surrendered" life is the militant, victorious life. Paul surrendered and Rome heard the gospel; Livingstone surrendered and Africa is turning to Christ; Huss surrendered and religious patriotism swept a nation; Luther surrendered and the Protestant Reformation shook the religious world. The Christian religion offers to the wills of men a great faith—a personal Christ as the supreme end of life. And this divine Leader announces, "And I, if I be lifted up, . . . will draw all men unto myself." Thus the selfish, discordant wills of men find themselves united in a harmonious and loyal service of the universal will.

Summary

The will is the mind's power to act. It is the personal self dominating its environment. It may act without conscious purpose; but it also acts in terms of future ends which it thinks are real and which can be fashioned by the act of willing. Smaller acts which are means to some larger purpose tend to become automatic. When the will ceases to be egoistic and loses itself in a larger personal end, it becomes faith; when it loses itself in an impersonal end, it becomes belief. The Christian religion provides a divine Person for the faith of all men. This Person is the Way, the Truth, the Life.

Questions for Review and Discussion

1. Define will, faith, belief.
2. Describe the two kinds of will.
3. Name three qualities which characterize the ends which the will chooses.
4. Give two simple rules for training the will.
5. Explain the difference between will and faith.
6. What is the quality which causes the "surrendered" life to be also the militant and victorious life?
7. What does the Christian religion furnish to the will?

LESSON VII
Habit Formation

Habit Defined. "Habit," said Dr. Emerson E. White, "is that which enables us to do easily, readily, and with growing certainty that which we do often." Every act leaves in the structure of the body and mind a capacity to repeat itself. There is a "set" of the mind and a "set" of the tissues of the body which make it easier for us to act in certain ways and harder to act in certain other ways. This **tendency to repeat** movements and thoughts is **habit**.

Value of Good Habits. Bad habits are our most persistent enemies. Good habits are our most helpful friends. Good and useful habits free the mind from the necessity of giving attention to many small details of conduct and enable it to devote itself to more serious and more important matters. One by one the mind hands the smaller duties over to the nervous system. At first, walking takes the entire attention of the child. Later, the child walks without thinking about it. Its nervous system is now able to attend to the whole walking process; walking is now a habit. Once we had to use our whole minds in order to shake hands with a friend; now we shake hands by means of our spinal cords, and our minds are free for more important matters. In like manner, we learn to do a multitude of things mechanically, habitually, with ease and accuracy, while our minds are struggling with problems that cannot be so easily reduced to habit and routine. Good habits thus insure economy and efficiency in our daily living. Our nervous system, trained to do many needful things for us promptly, efficiently, and certainly, comes to be the mind's most useful ally.

Kinds of Habits. Make a crease in a sheet of writing paper. At the line of the crease the fiber in the paper has taken on a new and modified form. The paper from now on tends to behave differently because of this changed structure of the creased portion of the paper. Inert, lifeless paper has a new habit!

Walk with "stooped" shoulders. Soon the living tissues of the body will adjust themselves to the "stooped" manner and you will be habitually "stoop-shouldered." Living tissues have acquired a "set," a habit of behavior. Of all living tissues the most delicate and sensitive is the nervous system. The play of color before the eye; the whisper of sound in the ear; the gentle touch of pollen from the rose in the nostrils; or the fleeting images of a daydream across the mind—all leave their indelible traces on the delicately attuned fibers of the nervous system. Every passing thought leaves its permanent tracing on the structure of the brain.

There are three ways by which habits are fixed in the nervous tissues: 1. **By repetition.** Every repeated act deepens the impression on the nervous system. 2. **By pleasurable associations.** If acts are associated with emotions that are pleasing, they will tend to be recalled more frequently and hence be more firmly fixed in consciousness. 3. **By acts of will.** If one gives conscious attention to impressions and by acts of the will recalls and reinstates them for the express purpose of making them automatic, the impressions are sure to be more deeply and more securely fixed upon the nervous system.

The Fateful Days of Youth. The delicate nervous system of the child is played upon by every wind that blows. The child must form habits. He is so made that **habits form themselves.** Habits of speech, of bodily carriage, of industry, of reading, of study—all are formed, for good or ill, in the days of youth. Schools are established and systems of training and discipline are created in order that these fateful days of youth, when the plastic organism is so keenly responsive, may be captured and used for the formation of good, useful, and permanent habits.

Habits the Schools Should Teach. The democratic state recognizes that people who are to live happily together in the same community must have certain common habits. These habits are or should be taught in the common schools. Among them are habits of communication: reading, writing; habits of coöperation: standing in line at a ticket window, carrying garbage to the garbage cans in order that the city may be clean, paying taxes, sharing common burdens and responsibility; habits of patriotism: saluting the flag, holding public office at personal loss to oneself; habits of industry; habits of recreation, et cetera.

Habits the Church Should Teach. There are certain essential habits which cannot be taught in the public schools. These habits must be taught by the schools of the church. Among them are habits of reverence: respect for the Sabbath Day; habits appropriate for God's house of worship; respect for God's Holy Book; habitual use of great hymns, prayers, Scriptures; habits of brotherly service; habits of honesty, truth-telling, personal cleanliness. The church school should coöperate with the public school in teaching such essential habits as obedience, promptness, helpfulness, and coöperation. Inaccuracy, disobedience, tardiness, carelessly prepared lessons, irregularity in attendance, are bad habits which the church school should strive to correct.

Rules for Forming New Habits. Professor James formulated three rules for establishing new habits: 1. "In the acquisition of a new habit, or the leaving off of an old one, we must take care **to launch ourselves with as strong and decided an initiative as possible.**" This means a vigorous beginning, with every condition arranged to favor the new and to discourage the old. A public pledge, a spectacular initiation, a new name or badge or costume, have their place in launching new habits. Greatly begin.

2. "**Never suffer an exception to occur until the new habit is securely rooted in your life.** Each lapse is like the letting fall of a ball of string which one is carefully winding up; a single slip undoes more than a great many turns will wind again. Continuity of training is the great means of making the nervous system act infallibly right." "Just

another cup to taper off on," said an old lady who was trying to break the coffee habit. The above rule indicates that "tapering off" is not the way to break a habit. There must be no exceptions. This being true, the Church should carefully nurture those who are striving to lead a new life. With high purpose they have "joined the Church." They have begun to lead a new life, but the old life of habit is still in their nervous systems. Their sins have been forgiven by a loving, heavenly Father, but their nervous systems have yet to be rebuilt so that they can fight a winning battle with the Adversary of their souls. Hence the new convert should be set to work at once, in helpful environment, and kept so constantly engaged in the new way of living that he will not "backslide," that there will be no chance to return to the old life until the reorganization of the nervous system in harmony with the new faith has rendered this return unlikely.

3. **"Seize the very first possible opportunity to act on every resolution you make, and on every emotional prompting you may experience in the direction of the habits you aspire to gain.** It is not in the moment of their forming, but in the moment of their producing **motor effects,** that resolves and aspirations communicate the new 'set' to the brain." (James, **"Brief Course in Psychology,"** p. 147.) With the mind constantly on the goal to be attained these three rules admonish us to (1) greatly **begin** (2) courageously **continue,** and (3) gloriously **achieve,** and lo, we have become new; old things have passed away and a new, redeemed self has, through God's help, come to be.

Summary

If we do not form habits they will form themselves. It is the law of our being. Good habits give us the constant and efficient help of our nervous system in achieving our ideals. Repetition, pleasurable associations, and conscious attention aid us in forming good habits. There are certain habits which should be taught in the public schools and there are certain other habits which should be taught by the Church. Three rules have been found helpful in breaking old habits and forming new habits.

Questions for Review and Discussion

1. Define habit.
2. State the value of good habits.

3. Name three ways to fix good habits in the nervous system.
4. Discuss the various kinds of habits.
5. What is the significance of youth for habit formation?
6. Enumerate habits which the public school should teach.
7. Enumerate habits which the church school should teach.
8. Discuss the three rules for breaking old habits and forming new habits.

LESSON VIII
How to Study

The Art of Study. The preceding chapter pointed out the importance of habit formation to the mental life. There is no more important habit than the habit of study. It is by the act of study that the subject matter of instruction is acquired and by this same act that valuable mental habits are formed. To learn to study efficiently is to acquire one of the finest of the fine arts. The importance of acquiring proper study habits is being more and more recognized in educational circles. Courses in supervised study are being provided in teachers' colleges and the literature of the teaching profession is giving careful attention to this subject.

The Conditions of Study. The most carefully formulated rules will be ineffectual if the conditions of study are not maintained. The body should be well, free from physical discomfiture. There should be freedom from fatigue. The blood should circulate freely and normally with no emotional obstructions within and no tight lacings or other restrictions without.

Unnecessary noise or disturbance should be removed. The study conditions should be pleasant, quiet, restful. One can study on trains, in shops, amidst the commotion of social gossip, but not efficiently.

Incentives to Study. The best student work is secured when the learner knows why he is learning this particular subject. The presence of an incentive or motive, immediate or remote, aids the student very greatly. When the pupil ceases to work for the teacher and begins to work for himself in order that he may achieve some worthy end through the results of study the efficiency of his work is immeasurably increased. It is a part of the task of the skillful teacher to present motives for study that will draw out the student's latent powers and secure the largest results through student interest and initiative.

Ten "Study Commandments." The psychological principles presented in earlier chapters of this book when applied to the mental processes involved in study give rise to the following rules:

1. **Maintain the conditions of study.** This applies to the student and his environment. Good health, fresh air, plenty of exercise, a quiet, restful place to study, freedom from eyestrain, proper temperature, and the like. The rasping voice of a scolding teacher or a nagging parent destroys attention and defeats the study process.

2. **Select a study place.** A certain room, a certain desk, a certain chair should be selected and used as a permanent study place. Instead of trying to study all over the house in all sorts of chairs and sofas, one place should be dedicated to study and nothing but study should be allowed in that place. Soon its very presence will suggest the study processes and the moment the student is seated in this particular place it will set the study processes going automatically.

3. **Select a study time.** A regular program of study should be made and followed. It is even desirable to set aside a particular hour for the study of each subject. The mind soon forms the habit of study at these particular times. It is not so important that the study time be morning, afternoon, or evening as it is that it shall be at **regular times**. In this connection it may be pointed out that there is no better discipline for a student than the practice of ordering his daily life in harmony with a fixed program of activity, which includes a certain hour for rising, another for meals, another for recreation, others for study and regular duties of the day, with a final time for retiring. The practice of beginning the day with a schedule of things to be done and a time devoted to each will make for habits of regularity and efficiency.

4. **Study hard while you are at it.** To the old adage, "Play while you play and work while you work," there should be added, "Study while you study." **Concentrate** from the first minute you begin to study. Let nothing interfere with your work. Do not worry or fret because you do not seem to learn fast. Keep clear-headed and cool, but just see to it that you do nothing else but study. If you must stop, do so at a logical break in your subject, and after a few minutes of relaxation come back to the work again. Make study a serious business.

5. **Consciously try to remember what you learn.** The student should say to himself, "I intend to remember this." Unless the learner tries to learn he will never learn. The very effort to learn sets a net

for ideas on the subject and presently the net is filled with ideas not only caught but partially digested. The preacher who selects his text on Monday morning will be surprised to find how many ideas have been caught by Friday morning when finally he begins to prepare his sermon. It is equally true with the student, who is learning any subject. Form the learner's attitude of mind and say, "I am learning this subject."

6. **Adopt a systematic method of study.** The following are suggested steps in the study of any lesson:

   (a) Briefly review the former lesson.
   (b) Make a preliminary survey of the assigned lesson.
   (c) Determine an order in which you will do the things required in this lesson.
   (d) Reserve most of your time for the hard points in the lesson.
   (e) Follow this plan until the lesson is learned.

7. **Memorize poems, orations, by "wholes" and not by "parts."** It is best to read such selections aloud, rapidly instead of slowly. The method of "wholes" may seem hard at first, but it will prove to be best.

8. **Make study periods long enough, but stop before you are fatigued.** It is best to study long enough at each time to get the advantage of the momentum one gains when once the study process is well under way.

9. **Outline the books, chapters, and lectures you hear and read and memorize your outlines.** The habit of selecting the leading topics in a lesson and logically organizing the material around a few main headings is a valuable aid to mental acquisition.

10. **Make some practical use of knowledge at the earliest possible moment after you learn it.**

Summary

Study is a fine art which can be learned. Proper incentives and proper study conditions are necessary. With these there remains only the willingness to follow certain simple "study commandments."

Questions for Review and Discussion

1. Discuss the importance of right study habits.
2. What are some of the conditions of study?
3. Enumerate some worthy study incentives
4. Repeat ten "study commandments."

LESSON IX
The Growing Mind

The Child Is Born a Human Being. From the instant of birth the baby is "dust of the ground" and "living soul." This wonderful combination of body and mind is a human being from the beginning. From the first moment the little mind is at work organizing its sense perceptions and preparing for the mental conquest of its environment. From the moment of birth there are the evidences of that trinity of power to **know**, to **feel**, and to **do**. But this **"immortal I,"** which we studied in Lesson I, must build up the content of its mental life through a long period of infancy. The fly has no period of infancy. From the moment of its birth it is prepared to perform all the duties of adult fly life, and it will grow to be just as big a fly and just as good a fly as either of its parents even though it never sees another fly. There are no fly nurseries and there are no fly academies just because there are no baby flies. But the human being has a long period of infancy during which to build up habits, ideas, and ideals with which to control its conduct through its mature life. The educator strives to put into the infant those controls, or methods and standards of conduct, which he would put into the race.

Child Study. The fact of infancy drives the educator to the study of the child. He knows the nature of consciousness, the structure of mind, and the anatomy and physiology of the adult body. He needs to know besides all these things the **laws of growth.** He needs to learn, for example, how memory develops in the mind of a baby in addition to the nature and laws of memory itself. General psychology, which deals with the analysis of the states of consciousness, needs to be supplemented by child psychology (generally called genetic psychology), which is concerned with the laws of mental growth. Upon general and genetic psychology the teacher builds his pedagogical methods.

Ten Periods in Human Development. The student of human development, while noting the almost imperceptible progress from infancy to maturity, finds it convenient to divide human development into "periods" or "stages" on the basis of the dominant physical and mental characteristics of the developing person. The following are the age groupings usually followed by the authorities in this field:

1. **The period of early infancy.** Ages, up to 3 years. A period of

beginnings in physical and mental life. The Cradle Roll period in the Sunday school.

2. **The period of later infancy.** Ages, 4 and 5 years. A period of rapid mental development and usually the period of the kindergarten and the Beginners Department of the Sunday school.

3. **The period of early childhood.** Ages, 6, 7, and 8 years. A period characterized by a rapid development of the imagination and the spirit of play and imitation. The Primary grades of the public schools and of the Sunday school.

4. **The period of later childhood.** Ages, 9, 10, 11 years. The pre-adolescent years. A period of rapid mental development and buoyant physical vigor. Sometimes known as the drill period. The intermediate grades in the public schools and the Junior Department of the Sunday school.

5. **The period of early adolescence.** Ages, 12, 13, and 14 years. A period of rapid physical growth. Self-consciousness again asserts itself. Mental life vigorous. The period of the junior high school and Intermediate Department of the Sunday school.

6. **The period of middle adolescence.** Ages, 15, 16, 17 years. A period of emotional development. Marked religious activity. The period of the senior high school and the Senior Department of the Sunday school.

7. **The period of later adolescence.** Ages, 18 to 23 years, inclusive. A period of rapid intellectual development. The period of logical analysis. This is the period covered by the college training and by the Young People's Department of the Sunday school.

8. **The period of early manhood and womanhood.** Ages, 25 to 34 years, inclusive. The period of new social, personal, and industrial or professional adjustments.

9. **The period of middle age.** Ages, 35 to 64 years, inclusive. This is the period which carries the load of mature life. Families are to be educated, business is to be developed, careers are to be made.

10. **The period of old age.** Ages, 65 years to death. This is a period of fruitage, of retirement, of wisdom, of devotion to worthy causes, depending on the ideals which have guided the earlier years.

Volumes could be written about each of these ten periods in the life of man. The parent and the teacher should be close students of the earlier periods especially, but those who are interested in the moral and religious life must not be neglectful of the later periods.

The Graded Church School. The graded public school is built to fit the needs of the graded child. Likewise the graded church school recognizes the needs of God's growing, developing, graded child. To meet the needs of the growing child there must, first of all, be a **graded curriculum** which will recognize the mental capacity of each period and provide materia for the religious training required by each period. In the second place, there must be a **graded organization** which will group children of the same ages together for special training, and make possible the special attention which each group needs. In the third place, there should be a **graded building and equipment**. The physical conditions in many churches are not adequate to meet the demands of efficient spiritual training of the children and youth of the parish. The problem of adapting the graded curriculum to schools of varying sizes, with partially trained leadership, is very difficult, but gradually the educators of the Church will solve this problem.

A Trained Leadership. The growing child demands a specially trained leadership. Experts, for example, must devote their lives to the problems of the religious training of children in early and later infancy. Literature must be developed, music prepared, training courses for parents prepared, and the whole program organized and promoted in such a way that there will be a revival of religious training in the home, and parents will be indeed the first religious teachers of their children.

What is true of the period of infancy is true of each of the other ten periods listed in this chapter. People must be set apart by the Church for this holy service and trained until they can render a significant service to the various areas of life to which they dedicate their talents.

There is a growing recognition of the demand for specialized leadership for the elementary grades and for the adolescent period, but there is not yet a definite recognition of the need for a study of the religious needs of adults as they pass through the states of adult experience. Men's Brotherhoods, adult departments in the Sunday school, and the like, which have been the recent attempts to care for these periods, have proceeded upon theories which did not adequately recognize the psychology of the mature mind and the religious needs of the different age groups in our adult life. This chapter pleads for a study of genetic psychology as well as for a study of general psychology by those who would direct the religious training of the boys and girls and the men and women of our churches.

Summary

The child is born a human being. He has a long period of infancy for growth and training. Racial progress depends in no small measure on the manner in which infancy is trained. Child psychology deals with the laws of mental growth. General psychology deals with the analysis of mind and its behavior. Both are needed by the educator. Ten periods have been designated as epochs or stages through which the human being passes from birth to death. The graded school is based upon these periods of development. The graded church school demands a specially trained leadership which can apply the laws of general and genetic psychology to the educational program of the Church.

Questions for Review and Discussion

1. Discuss the significance of human infancy.
2. Distinguish between general psychology and genetic psychology.
3. Name the ten periods of human development and give the age limits of each.
4. Explain how the graded church school is attempting to recognize these age groupings.
5. Name three things necessary to a graded school.
6. Discuss the need of a specialized leadership for religious schools.

LESSON X
Workers with Immortal Souls

A Trade or a Profession. Four elements enter into a trade or a profession, namely: **human needs, special knowledge, special tools,** and **craftsmanship** or **professional skill.** The shoemaker can have a trade so long as people wear shoes. To satisfy this need for shoes the shoemaker must have special knowledge about shoes, leather, lasts. He must also have special tools designed to aid in the work of making or mending shoes. Beyond this he must have skill in using the special tools and applying the special knowledge. If his motive in mending shoes is merely to make money for himself and he has no interest in developing his trade, he will have only a trade and he himself will be a mere artisan. But if he sees in his calling a worth-while method of serving his fellow men, and if besides mending shoes he develops new knowledge, perfects new tools, and acquires new skill for the good of his calling, he has become a craftsman—he has more than a trade; he has a **profession**.

A Classification of Occupations. If we were to classify the occupations of men on the basis of the character, quality, and intrinsic value of the raw material with which they work, we would have six groups or levels of workers. At the bottom of the list would be the **artisans** who work with brick and mortar, wood and stone, cloth and leather—workers with **inanimate matter**. Above the artisans would be the **engineers and machinists** who work with steam and electricity—with the **mysterious forces** of nature. This group satisfies human needs by the use of more refined knowledge, more complicated tools, and a higher type of skill than the group below. Next above the engineers are a group of **horticulturists** who work with **vegetable life**. They must master the secrets of life forces and coöperate with the laws of nature or their work will not succeed. Above the workers in vegetable life is the level of **animal husbandry** in which the raw material is **animal life**. These workers must master more complicated material than vegetable life. They must deal with more refined instruments of control. Above the level of animal life are the **teachers**, the educators who deal with **human consciousness**, who must master the laws which govern man's power to think and feel and do. And still above the teacher, at the very pinnacle of the vocational pyramid, are the **religious teachers and preachers** who deal with the **relation of the mind of man with the mind of God**.

All these groups are worthy callings. All satisfy human needs; all must have special knowledge; all must have special tools; and all must have a high degree of skill; but the first four deal with forces and substances that are finite and temporary and material, while the last two work with **the immortal souls of men**.

Sources of Knowledge of Mind. The teacher or religious worker who finds himself or herself custodian of the immortal souls of children or adults may wish guidance into the literature of this subject. These brief chapters have attempted only to introduce the reader to the field, to create a desire for future study and to create a sense of the dignity and majesty and sanctity of that **"immortal I"** which thinks and feels and wills.

The following books are recommended for future study:

Betts, George H., "The Mind and Its Education." Valuable for its simple treatment and its discussion of the physiological background of the mental life.

James, William, "A Briefer Course in Psychology." A classic which should be owned by every teacher.

Calkins, Mary W., "A First Book in Psychology." More technical than the preceding books. Contains most excellent chapters on Religious Consciousness.

Tracy, Frederick, "The Psychology of Childhood" and "The Psychology of Adolescence." Two valuable books on genetic psychology.

Whipple, Guy M., "How to Study Effectively." A little manual which should be owned by every teacher and by every high-school and college student.

Kitson, Harry D., "How to Use Your Mind." A more comprehensive treatment of how to study than Whipple's manual.

Religious Education as a Profession. There is no need to offer proof that religious education seeks to satisfy a fundamental need. There is rapidly being assembled, to satisfy this need, a body of specialized knowledge dealing with the religious training of children and adults. Gradually there is being developed a body of technical instruments, score cards, tests, and the like, which are the tools of this profession, and men and women are now in demand who can use these tools and apply this knowledge to the minds of children and youth. Yes, religious education is rapidly becoming one of the most important of the learned professions.

Builders of Ideals. Under the second heading in this chapter we classified the occupations of men on the basis of the kinds of raw material used. We pointed out that the two groups at the top work with the immortal souls of men. It now remains to call attention to the fact that teachers and religious workers furnish the **ideas and ideals** which all the other groups use. It is ideas and ideals that hold society together. Without them there could be no civilization and there would be no demand for other types of workers. It is teachers and religious leaders who weave ideas and ideals into the fabric of human experience and thus preserve our social institutions. The missionaries who have woven the ideals and ideas of the Holy Bible into the nations of the earth have laid the groundwork for a brotherhood of men.

In this age of materialism, in the aftermath of a great World War, young men and women are flocking into the four lower groups of occupations and there is great danger that there will not be enough workers in the upper groups to weave the warp of ideas and ideals which will hold civilization together. Many a time in the history of the world the warp has not held, civilization has collapsed, a period of dark ages ensued, and the mind of man has been compelled slowly to struggle up again through long centuries. Is history to repeat this catastrophe? It all depends upon the supply of ideas and ideals. Just now a clarion call is going out to the youth of the world to dedicate themselves to the upper levels of ideas and ideals. Upon the response to this call depends the civilization of the world. This whole book is a ringing challenge to you, reader, to dedicate your life to the higher levels and **become a worker with the souls of men.**

Summary

Every calling or profession seeks to satisfy the needs of men. Some occupations deal with material and temporal needs; other occupations deal with mental and spiritual needs of men. Civilization depends on the preservation of ideas and ideals; and these depend on a generous supply of men and women in each generation who dedicate their lives to the service of the higher needs of men. The present crisis in the world's history has produced a shortage of spiritual leaders, and civilization is now in danger of a complete collapse. The only hope for the present civilization is an army of volunteers for the service of ideas and ideals.

Questions for Review and Discussion

1. Name four elements which enter into a trade or profession.
2. Classify occupations on the basis of the raw materials used.
3. Name a half dozen books which will tell you more about the mind of man.
4. Show that religious education possesses all the elements of a profession.
5. Discuss the place of ideas and ideals in society.
6. Discuss the present need for religious teachers, preachers, missionaries, and social workers.

www.ingramcontent.com/pod-product-compliance
Lightning Source LLC
LaVergne TN
LVHW041510070426
835507LV00012B/1470